BULLETPROOF
YOUR SHOULDER

**Optimizing Shoulder Function to
End Pain and Resist Injury**

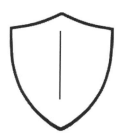

by

Jim Johnson, PT

This book was designed to provide accurate information in regard to the subject matter covered. It is sold with the understanding that the author is not engaged in rendering medical, psychological, or other professional services. If expert assistance is required, the services of a professional should be sought.

Drawings by Eunice Johnson

Published by Gatekeeper Press
2167 Stringtown Rd, Suite 109
Columbus, OH 43123-2989
www.GatekeeperPress.com

ISBN: 9781642376500
Library of Congress Control Number: Applied For

Printed in the United States of America

I have given my best effort to ensure that this book is entirely based upon scientific evidence and not on intuition, single case reports, opinions of authorities, anecdotal evidence, or unsystematic clinical observations. Where I do state my opinion in this book, it is directly stated as such.

—Jim Johnson, P.T.

WWW.BODYMENDING.COM

TABLE OF CONTENTS

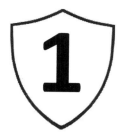

How to Bulletproof a Shoulder

Having a "bulletproof" shoulder is just a fun way of saying that you have a shoulder that is *pain-free* and *resistant to injury*. If you look around, you probably won't have to search too long to find someone with shoulder pain. Practically everyone has experienced it at one time or another, and for many, it never completely goes away. So just how does one go about "bulletproofing" their shoulder from pain and injury?

Bulletproofing From Pain

Tackling shoulder pain is not hard if you go at it with the right approach. Every time someone with shoulder pain comes to see me, I keep one thought in the back of my mind – the pain is most likely the result of something not functioning properly. My job as a physical therapist, then, is not necessarily to come up with the exact cause of someone's pain, *which can often times be either elusive or controversial*, but rather to figure out what the shoulder *isn't* doing that it normally should do. Using this approach during my evaluation, I routinely test the various shoulder functions – such as how strong certain muscles are or how far a patient can rotate their shoulder – so I can then determine what is or is not working up to par. Then, once the improper function has been identified, I can then choose a treatment that will restore it.

Consider the following list of possible treatments for shoulder pain...

- ice packs
- massage

- arthroscopy
- trigger point therapy
- whirlpool
- electrical stimulation
- mind-body techniques
- joint aspiration/injections
- heat
- total shoulder replacement
- range-of-motion exercises
- strengthening exercises
- pain medicines

As you can see from this rather lengthy list, medicine has come up with quite a wide range of treatment options when it comes to solving the problem of shoulder pain – and I'm sure there will be many more to come as time goes on.

While at first glance some of them appear to be *very* different from others, they all have a common thread running through them – *each of them is designed to restore or enhance the functioning of the shoulder area.*

Take a minute and think about it. Ice reduces swelling in your shoulder so you can raise it easier - and in turn it hurts a lot less. Strengthening exercises provide stability to the shoulder by making the muscles stronger. The most radical treatment of all, total shoulder replacement, improves the function of the entire shoulder area by putting in a new joint that can rotate and flex with ease.

Thinking about treating shoulder pain in this manner can be quite useful when one is trying to figure out what to do about it. As an example, if a shoulder is unable to rotate as far as it should, then a treatment is needed that will improve the shoulder's range of motion. And if one of the shoulder muscles were found to be weak, then a strengthening exercise would be in order. These, then, are the underlying principles this book will use to eliminate any existing shoulder pain you might have...

> Most shoulder pain is the result of dysfunction. Restore the function with the proper treatment and the pain will be relieved.

Another important point. Having treated shoulders for over twenty-three years, it's good to be aware of one common pitfall that's easy to fall into when trying to get rid of shoulder pain – focusing too much on structural abnormalities. What do I mean by *structural abnormalities*?

Well, here I'm talking about things like bone spurs, worn down cartilage, etc. Now it's not that they're insignificant and can't cause pain, *it's just that many people have them and have no pain* – so it's best to concentrate on restoring your shoulder function first - and then see where you're at. Here are some examples using one common structural abnormality you've probably heard of, the torn rotator cuff...

- one study did ultrasound scans on 237 people with *no shoulder pain* (Kim 2009). 41 of them had a torn rotator cuff in *at least* one shoulder. Interestingly, 4 had full-thickness tears (torn completely through) in *both* shoulders.

- an even larger study took 411 people with *no shoulder pain* (Tempelhof 1999). Ultrasound scans found torn rotator cuffs in 23% of subjects. Some of the tears were even massive, measuring over 5 centimeters long!

- MRI scans have found the same thing too (Sher 1995). One study looked at 96 subjects with *no shoulder pain*. How many had tears? A whopping 34%.

- this MRI study found that out of 100 people with *no shoulder pain*, 22 had partial rotator cuff tears and 14 had complete tears (Needell 1996). But what makes this investigation so interesting is the fact that they looked at the bones too. What else did they find in these subjects with no pain? 76% had some degree of shoulder arthritis, and 37% had bony spurs! Remember, these people had *no* shoulder pain at all.

- Ever hear of someone having a torn labrum? The labrum is a ring of cartilage in your shoulder joint that helps the shoulder bones fit together better. A 2011 study conducted ultrasound scans of 51 men with *no shoulder pain* – and found 14% had labral abnormalities (Girish 2011).

As you can see, there are a lot of people walking around with some pretty bad rotator cuff tears (and a slew of other abnormalities too), yet have *no pain* - which leaves us a little empty-handed at times trying to explain what exactly causes one's shoulder pain.

On the other hand, if you dig into the research on shoulder pain and *function*, you'll get a little different perspective on things. Here again, by function, I'm talking about how well a shoulder works and performs. Check out this study...

- there were 98 people with rotator cuff tears that had *no* shoulder pain

- these were compared to 62 people with rotator cuff tears *who had shoulder pain*

- researchers found no difference in the size of rotator cuff tears between the two groups

- researchers did, however, find more excessive motion in the group that had rotator cuff tears *and pain* (Keener 2009)

So here we have two groups of people with rotator cuff tears. One group has pain, and the other doesn't. If you just looked at the structural abnormalities, the tears, you wouldn't be able to tell who had shoulder pain and who didn't, because both groups had the same size tears. *On the other hand*, if you looked at who had the most extra motion in their shoulder joints, well, you *would* be able to predict who hurt and who didn't!

Hmm. Apparently there are *other* problems going on when one has shoulder pain other than just the structural abnormalities we see pictured all so clearly on MRI's and ultrasounds - problems such as excessive motion or weak muscles.

The point? If you have shoulder pain, and find you have a torn rotator cuff, arthritis in the joint, or other structural abnormalities such as these, don't panic and feel like all is lost. It is *quite* possible to have a structurally less than perfect shoulder, yet still feel just fine - so these "normal abnormal findings" might not necessarily be the cause of your pain. That's why it's so important to focus on improving the *function* of your shoulder first (after seeing a doctor of course), and address any structural abnormalities later on - if ever.

Bulletproofing from Injury

As we talked about earlier, having a bulletproof shoulder means having a shoulder that is pain-free and resistant to injury. Getting pain-free is a matter of treating anything that is not functioning properly in your shoulder and getting it up to par. So what's the plan for becoming resistant to injury?

Well, injury many times involves getting into a situation by chance. One example is falling down. Sometimes we just slip or trip, and reflexively reach out with our arm to break the fall – and injure the shoulder. Other examples are accidents that happen while lifting weights or playing a sport.

It's here that there's some good news and some bad news. The bad news is that there's not much you can do about chance occurrences or accidents most of the time – short of "just being careful". The good news, however, is that there is something you can do to eliminate, or at the very least *minimize* your chances of getting hurt when such unlucky events do occur – make sure your shoulder is *optimally functioning*.

That's right, we're back to the idea of improving shoulder function again. Just as improving shoulder function can get rid of pain, it can most certainly build a shoulder quite resistant to injury. In other words, a shoulder that has these four abilities can take a lot of abuse…

- ✓ **Superior Joint Stability**
- ✓ **A Rock-Solid Base**
- ✓ **Optimal Flexibility**
- ✓ **Finely-Tuned Proprioception**

The remainder of this book will go into great detail as to how you can quite easily develop each of the four abilities listed above that are absolutely essential to get a 100% optimally functioning shoulder, or in other words, a *bulletproof* shoulder. The following is a diagram that summarizes the concepts in this chapter that will be used in the pages that follow...

A normally functioning, pain-free shoulder possesses four abilities:

- good joint stability
- a solid base
- optimal flexibility
- intact proprioception

↓

Trauma, accidents, and aging changes

↓

Loss of Function

Shoulder loses one or more of the four abilities:
joint stability, solid base, optimal flexibility, finely-tuned proprioception

↓

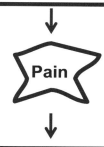
Pain

↓

Regain lost function by doing specific exercises to restore the four abilities

↓

The *Bulletproof* Shoulder
Pain-free – Resistant to Injury

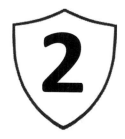

STEP ONE: CREATING A HIGHLY STABLE JOINT

When bulletproofing your shoulder, we're going to start with the very inside - the joint itself. Because some readers might not know how the shoulder is put together, it's best to briefly cover this first.

The Shoulder Bones

Let's get started with a basic picture of the bones that make up the shoulder area...

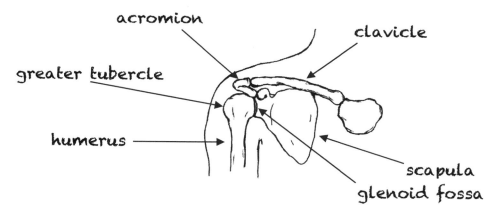

Figure 1. Looking at the right shoulder from the front – the bones that make up the shoulder area.

As you can see, the shoulder is made up of many different bones, most with some pretty odd shapes. While they're all important in one way or another, we really need to be concerned with just *three* of them.

The first one is known as the *humerus*, which is just a "funny" name for your upper arm bone. If you take another look at the above picture, you will notice a bumpy area at the end of it that bulges out. This particular part is known as the *greater tubercle*. You will find out shortly why this "big bump" is so important, but for now, just think of it as a hunk of bone that sticks out.

Next up we have the *scapula*, or what most people call their shoulder blade. The scapula is basically a triangular shaped bone with a couple of fingerlike projections poking out of one end. Pay particular attention to the one named the *acromion process* and the fact that is sits right over the humerus. Also notable is the *glenoid fossa*, which is a circular "crater" or socket that the humerus fits neatly into.

And last but not least, there's the *clavicle*, known to most of us as the collarbone. Oddly enough, it is the only bony connection between your arm and shoulder and the rest of your skeleton.

Although bones have many different functions, such as making blood cells and protecting vital organs, be aware that one of their main jobs is to provide firm places for the muscles to attach to.

The Shoulder Joints

Ever remember singing that song as a child, the one that goes "The foot bone's connected to the ankle bone..."? I'm betting most readers could still hum a few lines.

The point of this fun tune is that all the bones in our body are connected to each other and make up one big skeleton. In medical terms, the spot where two bones come together is known as a *joint*, and in the shoulder area, there are two important ones we need to talk about – the *glenohumeral joint* and the *acromioclavicular* joint. On the next page is an up-close look at them...

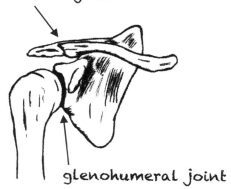

acromioclavicular joint

glenohumeral joint

**Figure 2. Looking at the right shoulder from the
front - the glenohumeral and acromioclavicular(A/C) joint.**

As you can see in the picture, the glenohumeral joint is where the *glenoid* fossa of the scapula bone meets the *humerus* bone, hence the name glenohumeral joint. And because the end of the humerus looks a lot like a ball, and the end of the scapula looks a lot like a socket, many people refer to this type of joint as a *ball and socket* joint. True to their shape, ball and socket joints can quite easily rotate in many different directions, which in turn allows us to move our arms and legs all over the place.

Now the other joint you'll need to be aware of is called the *acromioclavicular joint* or *A/C joint* for short. In keeping with all the other joint names, the A/C joint gets its tongue-twisting title from the fact that it is formed by two bones, the *acromion process* of the scapula (or shoulder blade) and the *clavicle* (or collarbone). Noteworthy because it sits right *above* the rotator cuff, the A/C joint too can dislocate, and when this happens, it is known as a *separated shoulder*.

The Best Way to Stabilize Your Shoulder Joint

From the above discussion, you know that you have two joints in your shoulder that allow movement, the glenohumeral joint and the acromioclavicular joint. While they're both important to overall shoulder movement, the crucial one to make as stable as possible is the glenohumeral or ball and socket joint. So why is that?

The short answer is because it's just not very stable to begin with. While you do have other ball and socket joints in your body, the shoulder's glenohumeral joint is just a little bit different. For comparison's sake, take a look at a picture of your right hip joint, which is also a ball and socket type joint...

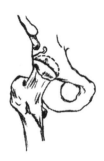

Figure 3. Looking at the right hip joint from the front – a deep ball and socket joint.

Now glance back at *the shoulder's* ball and socket joint in Figure 1. See any differences? I'll bet you do, an obvious one being that the hip joint has a fairly *deep* socket, while the shoulder joint a pretty *shallow* one. Unfortunately, from a mechanical standpoint, this brings both good *and* bad news for our shoulders.

On the upside, the shoulder *is* able move around freely in many more directions than most of the other joints in your body such as the hip. This is simply because a shoulder "ball" can move quite easily in its *shallow* socket than the hip's "ball" can in its *deep* socket. But on the downside, all this great motion comes at a price, that being that it leaves the shoulder *very* vulnerable to slipping out of alignment – which is where a lot of shoulder problems begin.

As an example, researchers have found that even when the ball part of the joint slips only a few millimeters out of it's place, it's linked to shoulder problems (Deutsch, 1996). And, looking at the other end of the spectrum, it's not uncommon to hear of the ball coming *completely* out of its socket and dislocating, as in the case of a person falling to the ground with an outstretched arm. Either way, the fact of the matter is that when it comes to the shoulder's ball and socket joint, it's definitely a case of Mother Nature trading *stability* for *mobility* – which is why we need to make this joint as stable as we possibly can. And how are we going to do that?

Well, we know there's nothing we can do about the way the bones fit together so shallowly. And then there are the ligaments, a tough tissue which connects and holds the bones together – they provide stability to the ball and socket - but there's not much you can do to drastically change their structure either. So that leaves *the muscles*.

Now we have something to work with. Muscles pull on the the bones to move and control their direction – and can help hold them in safe positions. By making the muscles a lot stronger, then, we've got more stability. In fact, the stronger you can make the muscles, the more shoulder joint stability you're going to have. Perhaps even better news, is that, while you've got a lot of different shoulder muscles, some are clearly more important than others, and there are only *a few* key muscles you've got to make stronger in order to gain super stability. And which ones would those be you ask?

The Rotator Cuff

A lot of people have heard of the rotator cuff, but my guess is most people don't *really* know exactly what it is or where it is. To begin with, there's the rotator cuff, which is actually made up of tendons, and then there's the rotator cuff *muscles* that are attached to them. Take a look...

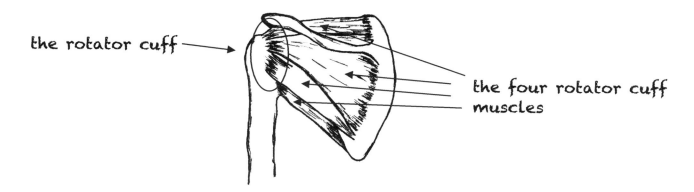

**Figure 4. Looking at the left shoulder from behind–
the rotator cuff and the rotator cuff muscles.**

As you can see, there are several arrows, one pointing to the rotator *cuff* and the others to the rotator cuff *muscles*. Although many people have a tendency to lump *all* of these structures together when they use the term "rotator cuff," know right off the bat that the rotator *cuff* is an entirely different kind of structure and tissue than the rotator cuff *muscles*.

The truth of the matter, and what a lot of people miss, is that the rotator cuff itself is really just a group of four flat **tendons** that fuse together and form a kind of "cuff" around the top part of your humerus. Since tendons connect the muscles to the bones, it's the job of the rotator cuff to help attach the rotator cuff muscles to the humerus. If any of this sounds a bit confusing, just remember that muscle connects to tendon, and tendon connects to bone - just like links in a chain. And the rotator cuff is *all* tendon.

The Rotator Cuff Muscles

If you counted them up in Figure 4, you found that there are no less than *four* rotator cuff muscles. Like the shoulder bones, scientists have also given the muscles some unusual names. They are:

- the supraspinatus
- the infraspinatus
- the teres minor
- the subscapularis

Clever readers will note that if you take the first letter of each muscle name and put them all together, they will actually spell out the word "SITS" – a little trick that has helped many a physical therapy student remember them all on test day.

Now since most of the rotator cuff muscles are pretty different from one another, and each have their own specific jobs, it's probably best if we take a brief look at them one by one.

Rotator Cuff Muscle Number One:
The Supraspinatus

Known for being the most frequently torn of all the rotator cuff muscles, the supraspinatus can be found on the *back* of your shoulder blade. It is here that it runs along the very top of this triangular bone and makes a straight shot to the greater tubercle, that "big bump" on your upper arm bone I pointed out earlier. Because it is buried under another muscle, as well as a bony part of the shoulder blade, it is hard to touch directly.

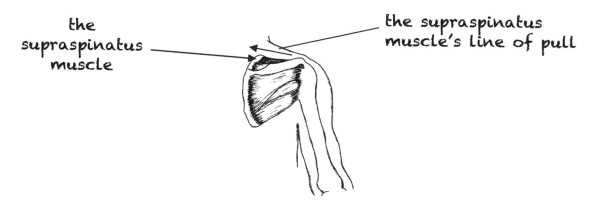

Figure 5. Looking at the right shoulder blade from the back – the supraspinatus muscle and its line of pull.

So what does the supraspinatus do anyway? Well, in order to figure out a muscles's function, researchers often look at what's called the "line of pull" of a muscle. Simply put, muscle fibers run in long, straight lines and pull on the bones when they contract By looking at the exact direction that they pull in, or their "line of pull," it can be determined which way a bone will move, the motion that will take place, and therefore what the muscle does. You can see the line of pull of the supraspinatus muscle represented by the top arrow in Figure 5.

Other clues can also be gotten by doing an *electromyographic* or *EMG study*. By inserting needles directly into the muscle of a subject and then asking them to move their shoulder around, the electrical activity of the muscle can be measured to see which motions the muscle is most active in.

Now as far as the job of the supraspinatus muscle, research has shown that its main task is to help you bring your arm out to the side, a motion referred to in medicine as *abduction*. Although the supraspinatus *is* very active in many other shoulder motions, abduction is considered its primary function.

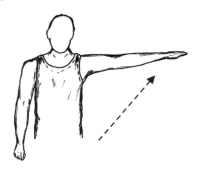

Figure 6. The supraspinatus muscle helps you raise your arm out to the side.

Rotator Cuff Muscles Two and Three: The Infraspinatus and Teres Minor

Figure 7 shows the next two rotator cuff muscles, the *infraspinatus* and *teres minor* muscles.

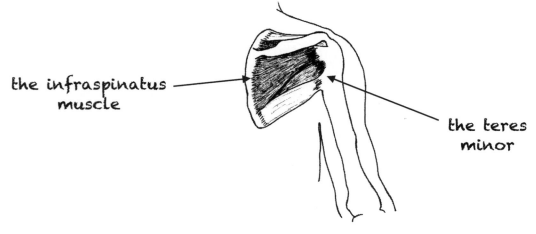

Figure 7. Looking at the right shoulder blade from the back – the infraspinatus and teres minor muscles.

As you can see, they sit right next to each other on the back of the shoulder blade. Because they both lie at the same angle and attach to the same area on the upper arm bone, they share the same job – to rotate your arm and shoulder *away* from your body. This motion is known as *external rotation*.

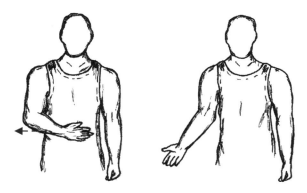

Figure 8. The job of the infraspinatus and teres minor muscles are to rotate your arm and shoulder *away* from your body.

Rotator Cuff Muscle Number Four:
The Subscapularis

The biggest and strongest of all the rotator cuff muscles, the *subscapularis* can be found taking up the entire *front* of the shoulder blade.

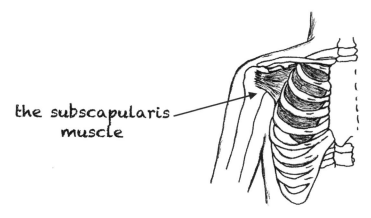

the subscapularis muscle

Figure 9. Looking at the right chest area from the front. The subscapularis muscle is located on the *front* of the shoulder blade

Like the teres minor and infraspinatus muscles, the subscapularis also helps you rotate your arm and shoulder around. However, instead of rotating them away from your body, the subscapularis is responsible for the exact opposite motion – rotating your arm and shoulder *towards* the body, a motion known as *internal rotation*.

The subscapularis gets this job because it attaches to the *front* of the upper arm bone, and not on the back, like the infraspinatus and teres minor muscles do. Here again, the spot where a muscle attaches to, as well as its line of pull, is very critical in determining what it will do.

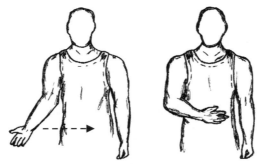

**Figure 10. The job of the subscapularis
is to rotate your arm and shoulder *towards* your body.**

Why the Rotator Cuff Muscles Are So Important

Up to this point you've learned that the majority of the rotator cuff muscles help with *rotating* the shoulder – which is of course how they got their name. But while we've covered what each *individual* muscle does, I have yet to tell you about their most important job – what they do when they all work *together*.

Remember when we said that the shoulder is a ball and socket joint that is very mobile, yet very prone to coming out of place due to its shallow socket? Well, although nature has put our shoulders at a slight mechanical disadvantage, it didn't leave us totally helpless either.

Instead of giving the shoulder a nice deep socket, like the hip joint, or lots of strong ligaments to hold the bones together, we've got the next best thing – powerful support from the rotator cuff muscles.

Individually, each of the four rotator cuff muscles have their own jobs. Some help roll the shoulder in, some help roll the shoulder out, and so on. But when all the rotator cuff muscles work *together* and contract at the same time, their combined pull helps keep the shoulder's ball and socket joint firmly in its place. Take a look at the line of pull of each individual rotator cuff muscle in Figure 11 and you'll see what I mean...

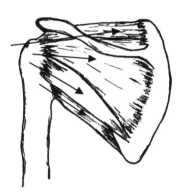

Figure 11. The lines of pull of the four rotator cuff muscles. When all of the rotator cuff muscles contract together, their combined forces hold the shoulder's ball and socket joint firmly in its place.

Each arrow in the above picture represents an angle that one of the four rotator cuff muscles is pulling in. As you can see, when the supraspinatus, infraspinatus, teres minor, and subscapularis muscles *all* contract at once, the net result is that the upper arm bone gets pulled snuggly towards the shoulder blade, thus firmly locking the "ball" into the "socket."

And when exactly does this happen, the rotator cuff muscles "kicking in" and contracting all at once to stabilize the shoulder joint? Well, according to the latest research, it occurs immediately *before* a person starts to move their shoulder around. For example, if you were to reach out right now and wave to someone, your rotator cuff muscles will contract the very instant *before* your arm actually starts to move. In this way, the shoulder joint starts out in a safe position and is held tightly in place as you go about using it. Pretty neat, huh?

Scientific-minded readers will also be glad to know that the research has definitely confirmed the stabilizing role of the rotator cuff muscles. A study published in the peer-reviewed journal *Clinical Biomechanics* involved recording the EMG activity of people's shoulder muscles as they were asked to perform certain motions (David, 2000). Sure enough, researchers found that a "pre-setting" of the rotator cuff muscles occurred before any shoulder motion actually took place. Other studies have found the same thing to occur (Day 2012).

The *Correct* Way to Get Your Rotator Cuff Muscles in Shape

Okay, now that we know that the key to gaining great shoulder joint stability is by strengthening the four rotator cuff muscles, it's time to learn *how*.

However before jumping right in and going over all the exercises you'll ever need to beef up your rotator cuff, I think it's best to begin with a few strength training basics. Because I wrote this book with *everyone* in mind – from the athlete, to the retired person who just wants to be able to lift up their grandkids – it's only wise to make sure that we're all on the same page before going any further.

Then, when we do get down to describing each of the strengthening exercises, *every* reader will know exactly what I mean when I say, "Do 1 set of 20 reps." So, using the handy question and answer format, let's start with the basics...

How do we make a muscle stronger?

Muscles get stronger only when we constantly challenge them to do more than they're used to doing. Do the same amount and type of activity over and over again, and your muscles will *never* increase in strength. For example, if Karen goes to the gym and lifts a ten-pound dumbbell up and down, ten times, workout after workout, week after week, her arms will *not* get any stronger by doing this exercise. Why? Because the human body is very efficient.

You see, right now, Karen's arm muscles can already do the job she is asking them to do (lift a ten-pound dumbbell ten times). Therefore, why should they bother growing any stronger? I mean after all, stronger, bigger muscles *do* require more calories, nutrition and maintenance from the body. And since they can *already* do everything they're asked to do, increasing in size and demanding more from the rest of the body would only be a waste of resources for no good reason.

It makes perfect sense if you stop and think about it, but we can also use this same line of thinking when it comes to making our muscles bigger and stronger – we simply *give* them a reason to get into better shape. And how do we do that? By simply asking them to do *more* than they're used to doing. Going back to the above example, if Karen wants make her arm muscles stronger, then she could maybe switch from a ten-pound dumbbell to a *twelve*-pound dumbbell the next time she goes to work out. Whoa! Her arm muscles won't be ready for that at all – they were always used to working with that ten-pound dumbbell. And so, they will have no choice but to get stronger now in order to meet the *new* demand Karen has placed on them.

For the more scientific-minded readers, the physiology textbooks call this *progressive resistance exercise.* You can use this very same strategy to get *any* muscle in your body stronger, and we're certainly going to be using it to get our rotator cuff muscles as strong as we can.

What's the difference between a repetition and a set?

As we've said, we need to constantly challenge our muscles in order to force them to get stronger, and one good way to do this is to lift a little heavier weight than we're used to using. Of course you won't always be able to lift a heavier and heavier weight *every* time you do an exercise, and so another option you have is to try to lift the same weight *more* times than you did before. As you can see, it's a good idea to keep track of things, just so you know for sure that you're actually making progress – which is where the terms "set" and "repetition" come into play.

If you take a weight and lift it up and down over your head once, you could say that you have just done one repetition or "rep" of that exercise. Likewise, if you take the same weight and lift it up and down a total of ten times over your head, then you could say that you did ten repetitions of that exercise.

A set, on the other hand, is simply a bunch of repetitions done one after the other. Using our above example once again, if you lifted a weight ten times over your head, and then rested, you would have just done one set of ten repetitions. Pretty straightforward isn't it?

Now the last thing you need to know about reps and sets is how we go about writing them down. The most common method used, is to first write the number of sets you did of an exercise, followed by an "x", and then the number of repetitions you did. For example, if you were able to lift a weight over your head ten times and then rested, you would write down 1x10. This means that you did 1 set of 10 repetitions of that particular exercise. Likewise, if the next workout you did 12 repetitions, you would write 1x12.

*What's the best number of sets and repetitions to do
in order to make a muscle stronger?*

There was a time when I asked myself that same question. So, in order to find out, I completely searched the published strength training literature starting from the year 1960. I then sorted out just the randomized controlled trials, since these provide the highest form of proof in medicine that something is really effective, and laid them all out on my kitchen table. While getting to that point took me literally months and months of daily reading and hunting down articles, it was really the only way I could come up with an accurate, evidence-based answer.

Now the first conclusion I came to was that it is quite possible for a person to get significantly stronger by doing any one of a *wide* variety of set and repetition combinations. For instance, one study might show that one set of eight to twelve repetitions could make a person stronger compared to a non-exercising control group – but then again so could four sets of thirteen to fifteen reps in another study.

Realizing this, I decided to change my strategy a bit and set my sights on finding the most *efficient* number of sets and repetitions. In other words, how many sets and repetitions could produce the *best* strength gains with the *least* amount of effort? And so, I had two issues to resolve. The first one was, "Are multiple sets of an exercise better than doing just one set?" and the second, "Exactly how many repetitions will produce the best strength gains?"

Anxious to get to the bottom of things, I returned once again to my pile of randomized controlled trials, this time searching for more specific answers. Here's what I found as far as sets are concerned:

- there are *many* randomized controlled trials showing that *one* set of an exercise is **just as good** as doing *three* sets of an exercise (Esquivel 2007, Starkey 1996, Reid 1987, Stowers 1983, Silvester 1982). This has been shown to be true in people who have just started weight training, as well in individuals that have been training for some time (Hass 2000).

Wow. With a lot of my patients either having limited time to exercise or just plain hating it altogether, that was really good news. I could now tell them that based on strong evidence from many randomized controlled trials, all they needed to do was just *one set* of an exercise to get stronger – which would get them every bit as strong as doing three!

And the best number of repetitions to do? Well, that wasn't quite as cut and dried. The first thing I noted from the literature was that different numbers of repetitions have totally different training effects on the muscles. You see, it seems that the lower numbers of repetitions, say three or seven for example, train the muscles more for *strength*. On the other hand, the higher repetition numbers, such as twenty or twenty-five, tend to increase a muscle's *endurance* more than strength (endurance is where a muscle must repeatedly contract over and over for a long period of time, such as when a person continuously moves their arms back and forth while vacuuming a rug for several minutes).

Another way to think about this is to simply imagine the repetition numbers sitting on a line. Repetitions that develop strength sit more toward the far left side of the line, and the number of repetitions that develop mainly endurance lie towards the right. Everything in the middle, therefore, would give you varying mixtures of both strength *and* endurance. The following is an example of this:

The Repetition Continuum

1 rep	10 reps	around 20 reps and higher

strength ————————————— endurance ————————➔

Please note, however, that it's not like you won't gain *any* strength at all if you do an exercise for twenty repetitions or more. It's just that you'll gain mainly muscular endurance, and not near as much strength than if you would have done fewer repetitions (such as five or ten).

Okay, so now I knew there was a big difference between the lower repetitions and the higher repetitions. However one last question still stuck in my mind. Among the lower repetitions, are some better than others for gaining strength? For example, can I tell my patients that they will get stronger by doing a set of three or four repetitions as opposed to doing a set of nine or ten?

Well, it turns out that there really is no difference. For example, one randomized controlled trial had groups of exercisers do either three sets of 2-3 repetitions, three sets of 5-6 repetitions, or three sets of 9-10 repetitions (O'Shea 1966). After six weeks of training, everyone improved in strength, *with no significant differences among the three groups.*

And so, with this last piece of information, my lengthy (but profitable) investigation had finally come to an end. After scrutinizing some 45-plus years of strength training research, I could now make the following evidence-based conclusions...

- ✓ **doing one set of an exercise is just as good as doing three sets of an exercise**
- ✓ **lower repetitions are best for building muscular strength, with no particular lower number being better than the others**
- ✓ **higher repetitions (around 20 or more) are best for building muscular *endurance***

In this book, we'll be taking full advantage of the above information by doing just one set of an exercise for ten to twenty repetitions. This means that you will use a weight that you can lift *at least* ten times in a row, and when you can lift it twenty times in good form, it's time to increase the weight a little to keep the progress going.

And why did I pick those numbers? Two reasons. The first has to do with the job of the rotator cuff muscles. Since they play a big role in stabilizing your shoulder, we want to boost their endurance and long holding time the most. And this means we're going to lean a little more towards the *upper* repetitions in order to boost the endurance ability of the rotator cuff muscles, while still staying low enough to substantially increase their strength. Remember, from around the twenty repetitions mark and up, you're going to gain mostly muscular endurance, and a lot less strength.

The second reason? Well, it's a matter of safety. Using higher repetitions enables us to not only gain plenty of strength, but also use much *lighter* weights than if we'd chosen to work with the lower repetitions. This is because it takes a much heavier weight to tire a muscle out in, say, five repetitions, than it does to tire a muscle out in fifteen. And since most people would agree that you have a better chance of injuring yourself with a heavier weight as opposed to a lighter one, I recommend leaning more towards the upper repetitions.

How many times a week do I have to do the exercises?

Doing the same strengthening exercise every day, or even five days a week, will usually lead to overtraining – which means *no* strength gains. This is because the muscles need time to recover, which typically means at least a day or so in between exercise bouts to rest and rebuild before you stress 'em again. And so, the question then becomes, which is better, one, two or three times a week?

Well, believe it or not, when I went through the strength training literature in search of the optimal number of times a week to do a strengthening exercise, there were a few randomized controlled trials actually showing that doing a strengthening exercise *once* a week was just as good as doing it two or three times a week. However, these studies were done on *very* specific populations (such as the elderly) or *very* specific muscle groups that were worked in a special manner. Therefore, when you take this information, and couple it with the fact that there are a few randomized controlled trials showing that two and three times a week are far better than one time a week, there really isn't much support for the average person to do a strengthening exercise once a week to get stronger. And so, we're again left with another question of which is better, two versus three times a week– which is what much of the strength training research has investigated.

However it is at this point that the waters start to get a little muddy. If you take all the randomized controlled trials comparing two times a week to three times a week, and lay them out on a table, you will get mixed results. In other words, there are some studies showing you that doing an exercise two times a week will get you the *same* results as three times a week, **but** there's also good research showing you that three times a week is *better* than two times a week. So what's one to do?

Well, in a case like this, the bottom line is that you can't really draw a firm conclusion one way or the other. So, you've got to work with what you've got. In this book, I'm going to recommend that you shoot for doing the strengthening exercises *three* times a week, because there is some good evidence that three times a week is better than two times a week (Braith 1989). However, I'm also going to add that if you have an unbelievably busy week, or just plain forget to do the exercises, I'll settle for two times a week because there is also substantial evidence that working out two times a week is just as good as working out three times a week (Carroll 1998, DeMichele 1997).

So there you have it. While it may have been a whole lot easier to just answer the question by saying "do the strengthening exercise two to three times a week," I think it's good for readers to know *exactly* why they're doing the things I'm suggesting *and* that there's a good, evidence-based reason behind it.

How hard should I push it when I do a set?

How hard you push yourself while doing an exercise, also known as *exercise intensity*, is another issue that certainly deserves mention and is a question I am frequently asked by patients. The answer lies in two pieces of information:

1. Doing an exercise until no further repetitions can be done in good form is called *momentary muscular failure*. Research shows us that getting to momentary muscular failure or close to it produces the best strength gains.

2. You should not be in pain while exercising.

Taking the above information into consideration, I feel that a person should keep doing an exercise as long as it isn't painful and until no further repetitions can be done in good form within the repetition scheme.

Does it make any difference how fast you do a repetition?

Many randomized controlled trials have shown that as far as gaining strength is concerned, it does *not* matter whether you do a repetition fast or slow (Berger 1966, Palmieri 1987, Young 1993). Here's a look at one of the studies:

- subjects were randomly divided into three groups (Berger 1966)
- each group did one set of the bench press exercise, which was performed in 25 seconds
- the first group did 4 repetitions in 25 seconds, the second group did 8-10 repetitions in 25 seconds, and the third did 18-20 repetitions in 25 seconds
- at the end of eight weeks, *there were no significant differences in the amount of strength gained between any of the groups*

So that's the evidence-based guidelines as far as strength is concerned. As far as safety, I recommend that you lift the weight up and down *smoothly* with each repetition, carefully avoiding any jerking motions.

What equipment will I need?

Since you'll be doing strengthening exercises that involve lifting a weight, it's a no brainer you're going to need something to lift. Remember from our earlier discussion that muscles get stronger only when we constantly challenge them to do more than they're used to doing. So, this means that taking the same weight, and lifting it over and over again, week after week, simply won't get the job done. Therefore, you'll need to have *several* weights of varying pounds available to use.

By far the easiest thing to do is to just go to a sporting goods store (or large retail store), and purchase several light dumbbells. Most look something like this:

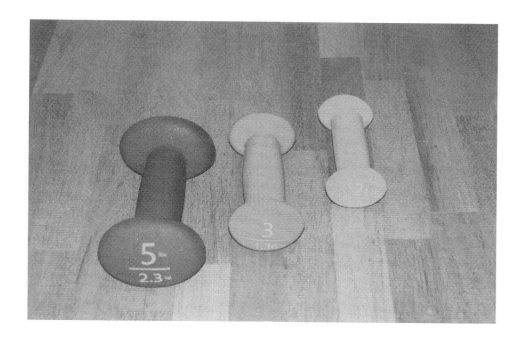

Light dumbbells such as these are inexpensive, which is a good thing, because you're going to need to get several different sizes as you progress and get stronger with the exercise program. Of course you technically can use any kind of weight that's comfortable to grip and allows you to progress to a heavier weight in small increments.

How much weight should I start off with?

For reasons we've discussed earlier in this chapter, I recommend you shoot for doing one set of an exercise for ten to twenty repetitions. Therefore, you should start out with a weight that allows you to do a minimum of ten repetitions, but no more than twenty. But how do you figure that out?

Well, by a little trial and error. The first time you do a particular exercise, you're just going to have to take your best guess at to how much weight will allow you to do between 10 and 20 repetitions, try the exercise, and then see how it goes. As an example, say you're going to try a rotator cuff exercise and decide to try two pounds, begin lifting it, and find you can do 15 repetitions in good form. That's great – you've hit our target range of 10 to 20 reps! Next time, you'll use two pounds again, and try and do a few more reps, eventually working up to 20 reps before adding more weight.

The other thing that commonly happens when you're doing an exercise for the first time, is that you might find it's either too heavy (maybe you could lift it only once or twice) *or* it's way too light (maybe you could lift it twenty-five times or more). Here again, that's not a big problem. When trying the exercise the next time, simply take another good guess and adjust the weight up or down a little as needed. Do keep in mind that when *anyone* starts a weight training program, or tries a new exercise for the first time, it's perfectly normal for it to take one or two exercise sessions to find the appropriate weight.

Like I said, it'll be a matter of a little trial and error at first, but do keep in mind that when it comes to strengthening your rotator cuff, the main idea is not to see how much weight you can lift, but rather to find a safe starting weight, and then *gradually progress* over time.

And with that last bit of strength-training information, we're finished discussing the basics. So, now that we're all on the same page, let's move on to some of the best rotator cuff strengthening exercises medical research has to offer...

Rotator Cuff Exercise #1:
~ Sidelying Abduction~
Works the Supraspinatus

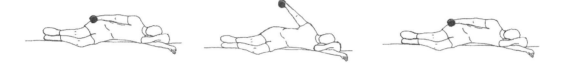

starting position   midpoint   finishing position

How to do it: First, get in a comfortable position on your side, making sure that the shoulder you are going to strengthen is the one *on the top.* Next, hold a dumbbell in your hand with your arm on your side like the far left picture. Now smoothly lift the weight up towards the ceiling, *going no higher than a forty-five degree angle* (as in the middle picture). Lower smoothly and repeat, working up to twenty times in a row, once a day.

Precautions: It's essential that you don't raise your arm up any higher than a forty-five degree angle when doing this exercise. Why? Going higher could cause impingement – which means pinching an irritated bursae or rotator cuff that is trying to heal.

Notes: This is one of the safest exercises you can do to strengthen your supraspinatus muscle – the most frequently torn of the four rotator cuff muscles.

It's a Fact!
The following published EMG studies have confirmed that the supraspinatus muscle is *highly active* when doing this specific exercise.

✓ **Wickham 2010, McMahon 1996**
✓ **Additionally, an MRI study, Horrigan 1999, has also shown this**

Rotator Cuff Exercise #2:
~Sidelying External Rotation~
Works the Infraspinatus and Teres Minor Muscles

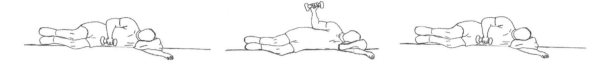

| starting position | midpoint | finishing position |

How to do it: First, get in a comfortable position on your side, making sure that the shoulder you are going to strengthen is the one *on top*. Next, hold a dumbbell in your hand with your arm bent ninety-degrees at the elbow like the above pictures. Now smoothly lift the weight up as high as you comfortably can, making sure that you keep the ninety-degree bend in your elbow. Lower smoothly and repeat, working up to twenty times in a row, once a day

Precautions: Make sure you're not rolling your body back as you do the exercise or lifting your *upper* arm off your body–it should stay on your side. Also, it's essential that you keep the ninety-degree bend in your elbow the entire time you're doing the exercise to make sure your rotator cuff is doing most of the work.

Notes: How high up you raise the weight towards the ceiling depends upon factors such as how irritated your shoulder might be, or how much tightness you have in your shoulder. Therefore, rather than worrying about raising your arm up to a set height, just concentrate on keeping your arm motion within a comfortable range. In time, chances are you'll notice that you will be able to lift your arm up higher and higher as your shoulder loosens up and becomes stronger.

It's a Fact!
The following published EMG studies have confirmed that the infraspinatus and teres minor muscles are *highly active* when doing this specific exercise.

✓ **Andersen 2010, Reinold 2004, Hintermeister 1998, Ballantyne 1993, Townsend 1991**

Rotator Cuff Exercise #3:
~Liftoff~
Works the Subscapularis Muscle

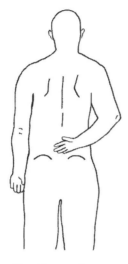

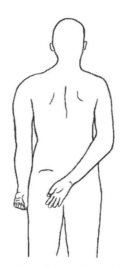

Preferred:
hand in small of back

For the less flexible:
hand lower down on buttock

How to do it: This exercise is done quite easily. To do it, you simply place your hand in the small of your back, in the middle. Then, you simply lift your hand **up off your back**. Repeat, working up to twenty times in a row, once a day.

Precautions: It's essential that you lift your hand straight off your back – avoid pulling it up, down, or side-to-side as you lift the hand up.

Notes: If you find it hard to place your hand in the small of your back, it is okay to place it lower down on the buttock, however doing it like this decreases subscapularis muscle activity by 30% (Greis 1996). Also, a small weight in the hand is used to increase resistance as needed.

It's a Fact!
The following published EMG studies have confirmed that the subscapularis muscle is *highly active* when doing this specific exercise.

✓ **Suenaga 2003, Greis 1996, Kelly 1996**

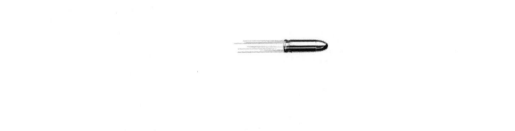

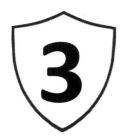

STEP TWO: BUILDING A SOLID BASE

If you only do the three exercises in the last chapter, you'll have created a *very* stable shoulder joint, that's for sure. Problem is, the shoulder joint works on a base of support, that being your shoulder blade, or *scapula*. Take a look…

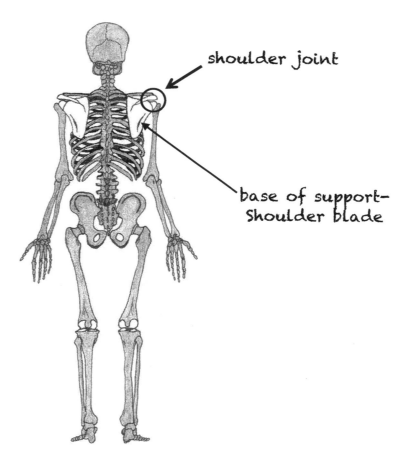

shoulder joint

base of support- Shoulder blade

Figure 12. Looking at the human skelton from behind
Note how the triangular shaped shoulder blade is the supporting
base for the shoulder *joint.*

You wouldn't build a house on sand, and you certainly don't want to build a stable shoulder joint on a weak base, the shoulder blade. In short, your shoulder's ball and socket joint needs a solid, stable base from which to work efficiently on.

Another thing most people don't realize about the shoulder, is that as you raise your arm, your shoulder blade moves as well. Let's take an X-ray look at what exactly is happening as you reach up for something...

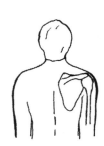 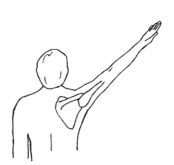 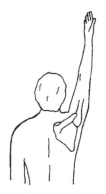

Figure 13. Looking at the right shoulder from the back. Note the resting position of the shoulder blade and upper arm bone.	**Figure 14. As the arm is raised, note that not only has the upper arm bone moved, but so has the shoulder blade. Can you see that the shoulder blade has tilted up as the arm was raised?**	**Figure 15. Look at the shoulder blade now as the arm reaches way up. Compare this to the shoulder blade's original resting position in Fig. 13.**

As you can see, reaching around and doing things involves a whole lot more than just your arm and shoulder joint. Because your upper arm bone or *humerus* is attached directly to your shoulder blade, the two move in harmony as you use your arm to do things in various directions. In physical therapy school, I learned that this interaction is called your *scapulohumeral rhythm*. It's kind of a tongue twister, but just remember that all it really means is that as your upper arm bone is raised up, the shoulder blade comes along with it to varying degrees.

Now that you have that bit of knowledge, you can now see that the shoulder blade is really the "base of support" for the shoulder's ball and socket joint – which is exactly where the shoulder blade muscles come in – they are supposed to keep the shoulder blade *precisely* where it's suppose to be.

Here's a list of the major muscles that move the shoulder blade around as well as stabilize it:

- the rhomboids
- the trapezius muscle
- the levator scapulae
- the serratus anterior

All these muscles attach directly to your shoulder blade, and when they are strong and doing what they're suppose to do, all is well – your shoulder joint has a stable base to work from - and the rotator cuff muscles can do their job too without problems.

If, however, your shoulder blade muscles are weak or tire easily, the shoulder blade can start to move around abnormally and stir up trouble. For example, abnormal shoulder motion has been found in one of the most common shoulder problems – *impingement syndrome* (McClure 2006).

Impingement Syndrome

At this point, most readers are probably thinking one of two things: "What the heck is impingement syndrome?" *or* "That's what I have!" In either case, I need to explain exactly what impingement syndrome is because I have known it to mean different things to different people. Sooo, let's start at square one.

When something is "impinged" it means that something is being squished between two things. If you've ever gotten your finger caught in a drawer or a doorway, your finger was being pinched or "impinged."

A similar thing can happen in the shoulder. This time, however, instead of your finger, it's your rotator cuff and a few other structures that can be pinched in an area known as the *subacromial space*. Here's where it's at:

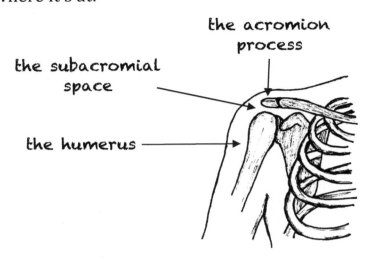

Figure 16 Looking at the right shoulder from the front – the subacromial space. In this space lies the rotator cuff as well as the subacromial bursa.

As you can see, the subacromial space is the area that lies *below* the acromion process, and *above* the humerus. Therefore, everything within this space sits right between two hard bones – which is precisely where the pinching or impingement can take place.

While many important structures can be pinched in the subacromial space, we're really concerned with just two in particular – the rotator cuff and something called *the subacromial bursa.* Since you're already a little familiar with the rotator cuff from the previous chapter, let's talk about the subacromial bursa for a moment.

Bursae in general are flat, sac-like structures that are located all throughout your body. If you've ever seen a deflated whoopie cushion, well, that's about what they look like. The shoulder's subacromial bursa is really no different than any of the other bursae, but since its home is right *below* the bony acromion process, it's called the *sub*acromial bursa.

Now it's the main job of these bursae to reduce friction and make things slide a whole lot easier, particularly in areas where structures have a tendency to rub together a lot – like when a tendon passes right over a bone. Normally they contain a small amount of fluid, however if they get irritated, they can really swell up and cause you a lot of pain. When this happens, doctor's call it *shoulder bursitis*, a condition I'm sure most readers have heard of before.

Having said all that, you now know what impingement is (something being pinched), where it takes place (the subacromial space), and what important structures get impinged (the rotator cuff and subacromial bursa). So, next we need to talk about *when* this problem can happen.

Figure 17 showns the subacromial space when your arm is hanging down at your side – a fairly good gap as you can see. Now take a look at Figure 18, which shows us what happens to the subacromial space *when you raise your arm up to use it.*

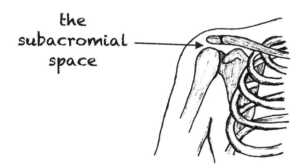

Figure 17. The subacromial space when your arm is hanging down at your side.

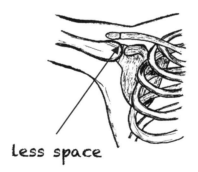

Figure 18. The subacromial space when you raise your arm up to use it.

Wow! As you can see, the subacromial space does *not* always stay the same size. In fact, it gets *even smaller* when you raise your arm up. And just why is that? Well, largely because of the greater tubercle, that big bump on your upper arm bone I told you about earlier. Raising your arm brings the greater tubercle up and into the subacromial space where it takes up more room in an already crowded area – thus contributing to impingement of the rotator cuff tendons and bursa that sit directly above it.

At this point though, I need to make it perfectly clear that just because the subacromial space gets smaller when you raise your arm, that does *not* mean that the poor little rotator cuff and bursa are being brutally pinched all the time. As a matter of fact, in a normal state, when everything in the shoulder is functioning as it should, there is just enough room for all the structures in the subacromial space to carry on just fine *without* being impinged. However since space *is* limited and things are packed in there rather tightly, there's not much room for error either. So, when things do get out of whack and pinching does occur, you have what is called *impingement syndrome*.

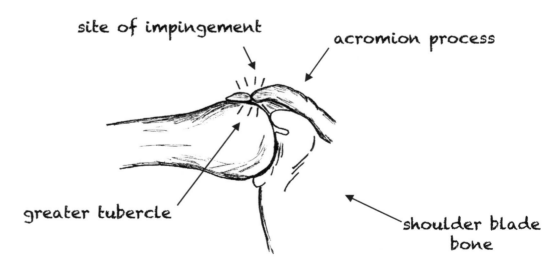

Figure 19. Looking at the right shoulder from the front. Impingement syndrome occurs when the subacromial bursa and rotator cuff get pinched between the acromion process and greater tubercle. This impingement happens as you raise up your arm.

Now besides impingement syndrome, a lot of research has found abnormal shoulder blade motion going on in *many other* different kinds of shoulder problems...

- people with unstable shoulder joints (Ogston 2007)
- people with shoulder pain and loss of shoulder motion (Lin 2005)
- rotator cuff tears (Paletta 1997)

In all these studies, researchers have taken the shoulders of subjects with various shoulder problems, and compared them to an asymptomatic control group using sophisticated systems to track shoulder blade motion to tell what's going on. Here's a closer look now at the muscles we mentioned earlier that you'll need to strengthen to build a solid base of support - and bulletproof yourself against all the shoulder problems we've just been talking about...

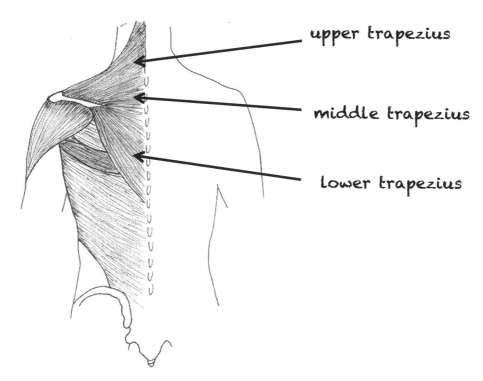

upper trapezius

middle trapezius

lower trapezius

Figure 20. The outer most layer of scapular stabilizers – the upper, middle, and lower trapezius. Notice that each part of the trapezius has it's own distinct fiber direction, and thus pulls the shoulder blade a little different direction.

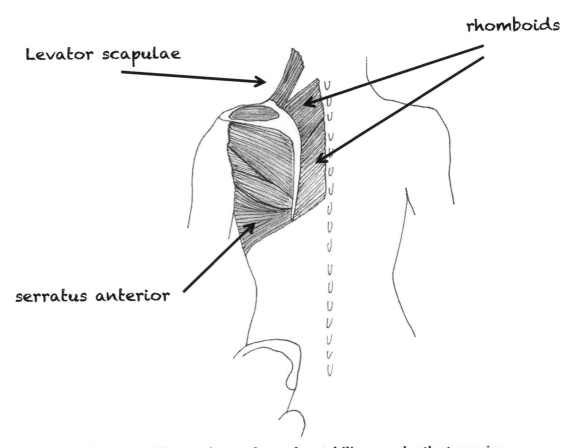

Figure 21. The next layer of scapular stabilizers under the trapezius –
the levator scapulae, rhomboids, and the serratus anterior. Again, each
muscle has a unique line pull allowing them to stabilize the shoulder
blade at many different angles.

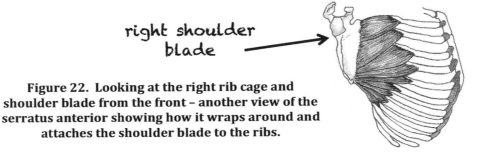

Figure 22. Looking at the right rib cage and
shoulder blade from the front – another view of the
serratus anterior showing how it wraps around and
attaches the shoulder blade to the ribs.

A lot of funny looking muscles with a lot of funny names – but all necessary as the shoulder blade is capable of moving in quite a lot of different directions...

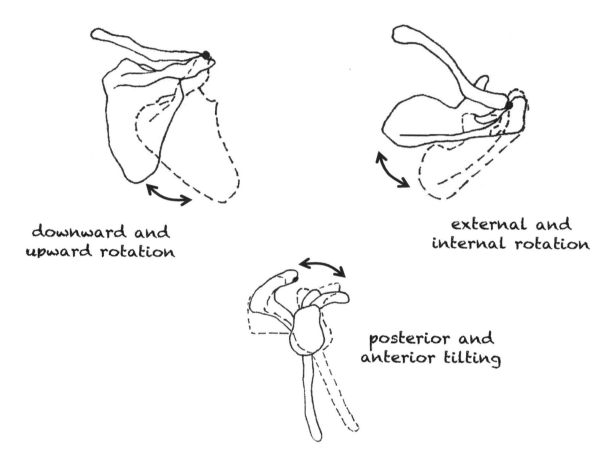

downward and
upward rotation

external and
internal rotation

posterior and
anterior tilting

**Figure 23. The many motions that a shoulder blade
is capable of as you move your arm around.**

In short, the shoulder's ball and socket joint sits on a *very* mobile base – making it a good idea to make this base as solid as possible. Does it take a lot of exercises to builds a rock-solid base of support? Nope, just two good ones...

Scapular Stabilization Exercise #1
~Rowing~
Works the Upper-Middle-Lower Trapezius, Rhomboids, and Levator Scapulae Muscles

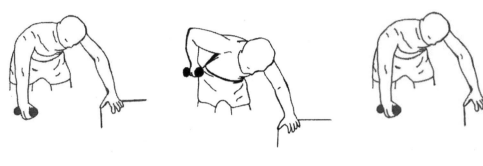

starting position   midpoint   finish position

How to do it: First, find a sturdy object to lean on, such as a table-top. Next, hold a dumbbell in the hand of the shoulder you want to strengthen, and get into the starting position (far left picture). Now smoothly bend your elbow and pull the dumbbell straight up to your side. Lower smoothly and repeat, working up to twenty times in a row, once a day.

Precautions: Make sure that you bend over approximately forty-five degrees like the above pictures. There's no need to bend over more than that, but if you're not bent over far enough, the shoulder blade muscles won't get worked adequately.

Notes: This one exercise works *many* of the muscles that control and stabilize your scapulae (shoulder blade).

It's a Fact!
The following published EMG studies have confirmed that the upper-middle-lower trapezius, rhomboids, and levator scapulae muscles are *highly active* when doing this specific exercise.

✓   Andersen 2012, Schachter 2010, Moseley 1992

Scapular Stabilization Exercise #2:
~ Sidelying Abduction~
Works the Serratus Anterior Muscle
(in addition to the Supraspinatus)

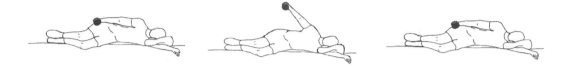

starting position   midpoint   finishing position

How to do it: First, get in a comfortable position on your side, making sure that the shoulder you are going to strengthen is the one *on the top*. Next, hold a dumbbell in your hand with your arm on your side like the far left picture. Now smoothly lift the weight up towards the ceiling, *going no higher than a forty-five degree angle* (as in the middle picture). Lower smoothly and repeat, working up to twenty times in a row, once a day.

Precautions: It's essential that you don't raise your arm up any higher than a forty-five degree angle when doing this exercise. Why? Going higher could cause impingement – which means pinching an irritated bursae or rotator cuff that is trying to heal.

Notes: Yes, you're not imagining things, this is the same exercise from the last chapter I gave you to strengthen your supraspinatus muscle. Because the serratus anterior muscle is so active in this particular exercise, we can also use it to strengthen the serratus anterior too!

It's a Fact!
The following published EMG studies have confirmed that both the middle and lower parts of the serratus anterior muscle are *highly active* when doing this specific exercise.

✓ **Parry 2012, Wickham 2010, Faria 2008, McMahon 1996, Moseley 1992**

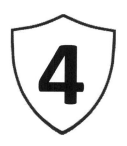

STEP THREE: DEVELOPING OPTIMAL FLEXIBILITY

So far we've talked about building a stable shoulder joint with a solid base of support. However, if you stopped there and just did those four exercises, you would *not* have a bulletproof shoulder. Why? Because the strongest, most stable shoulder in the world is practically useless if all it can do is move around a few degrees in each direction. While most of us can probably move are arms around fairly well, a bulletproof shoulder is one that has *optimal* flexibility in *all* the major directions – such as *external rotation*.

Why Your Shoulder Might Not Be As Flexible As It Should Be

Every reader will most likely have a slightly different amount of tightness in his or her shoulder. Some might not be able to put their hand behind their back very well, while others may have difficulty raising their arm up very high. The specific stretches in this chapter will help you restore all the major motions in your shoulder, getting it up to peak performance. But first, what is preventing your shoulder from moving freely in all directions?

Well, there are lots of reasons why people can lack flexibility in their shoulders, and no two readers may have the exact same cause. On the next page is a table that lists some common reasons why shoulder motion can be limited...

Problems that may lead to a loss of shoulder flexibility	Possible causes of this problem	Common Treatments
Swelling	Fluid in the shoulder joint that takes up space and prevents full motion	Ice, stretching, removal of fluid by needle, anti-inflammatory medications
Tight Muscles	Muscles become shorter when not regularly stretched through their full range of motion	Stretching exercises
Mechanical Problems	Problems such as torn cartilage or loose bodies in the joint can block normal motion between the bones	In some situations, surgical removal
Pain	A shoulder that hurts doesn't move through a full range of motion, causing muscles and other structures to shorten over time	Exercise, pain medications
Tight Joint Capsule	The tissue that surrounds the entire joint can become tight, keeping the bones from moving normally	Stretching, joint manipulation

You can see from the list that there are various causes of lost shoulder motion – and, likewise, various treatments to correct these problems. Although this is a do-it-yourself book, I would like to make it clear that not all cases can be treated conservatively at home. For instance, a person who has a loose body, such as a piece of torn tissue in his or her shoulder – a problem that can mechanically block shoulder motion much like a marble in a gearbox – could quite possibly need surgery. Realistically, though, most people with this type of problem will probably not be reading this book, but rather end up at the doctor's office, because it will be obvious that something major has gone wrong. Indeed, many readers with decreased shoulder motion can be more than adequately treated with a simple stretching program, done correctly. My only point here is to let you know that although stretching is indicated most frequently in the vast majority of cases, it is not a universal treatment. Please consult your medical professional should any questions arise.

Some readers may also have noticed that what is missing from the list of causes are specific ailments such as arthritis. That is because in this book we're more concerned with function rather than labels. Therefore, when looking at why a shoulder isn't able to be raised up fully, we don't say it's because of arthritis, but rather because of the pain, swelling, or muscle tightness that's secondary to arthritis. And why is it a good idea to think about it like this? Because doing so helps us better zero in on specific *functional* problems we can treat.

How Much Motion Should a Normal Shoulder Have Anyway?

A good question, as I just hate it when people are given stretches to do, but no clear guidelines as to when they need to stop. Let's first start out by looking at what is considered "normal" shoulder motion. Here's part of a list I compiled one time when I was looking into this matter:

source	shoulder flexion	shoulder external rotation	shoulder internal rotation
American Academy of Orthopaedic Surgeons (1965)	180°	90°	70°
Boone (1979)	167°	104°	69°
Esch (1974)	170°	90°	80°
Journal of the American Medical Association (1958)	150°	90°	40°
Kapandji (1970)	180°	80°	95°

As you can see by all the different numbers, there certainly seems to be a lot of confusion over what is considered "normal" shoulder motion. And why is that? Well, if you scrutinize the studies closely as I have, the answer becomes obvious. Some studies measured *young* subjects, some *older* subjects, and some measured just *male* subjects. And to further complicate things, not all studies were even using the same method of measurement. No wonder it's so hard to sort things out! So, what do we do now?

Well, research was done once that measured four major shoulder motions in eighty-one normal subjects, aged 60 to 70 years of age, and calculated their average flexibility (Matsen, 1994). Therefore, given that you're not much over 70, I'm thinking that this would be a good *minimum* amount of shoulder motion for most readers to shoot for. After all, if a group of senior citizens have this much motion in their non-problematic aging shoulders, it's not unreasonable to expect that people younger than this should *at least* be this flexible.

Now the four major shoulder motions tested in this study were flexion, external rotation, internal rotation, and horizontal adduction. Since some of these motions I haven't explained and probably sound funny to most readers, here are some pictures showing each motion, how it's measured, as well as how much motion you should probably have as a minimum. Here they are...

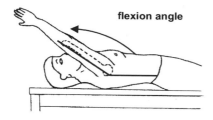

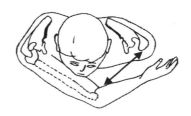

Motion: flexion
Minimum flexibility: 160° for males
167° for females

Note: A 0° angle would be lying on your back with your arm at your side, a 90° angle would be your arm pointing straight up to the ceiling, and a 180° angle would be when your arm is over your head and parallel to the floor. You can estimate your flexibility from these points. Get the help of an observer if you need to.

Motion: horizontal adduction
Minimum flexibility: 15 cm for males
14 cm for females

Note: Horizontal adduction is measured as the distance between your inner elbow and the bony bump on the front part of your shoulder (the acromion process). Use a tape measure and grab a buddy to get this measurement.

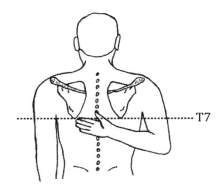

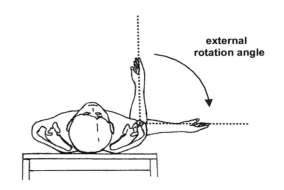

Motion: shoulder *internal* rotation
Minimum flexibility: T6 for males
                             T5 for females

Note: The T7 level is approximately the bottom tip of your shoulder blade. T6 is about 1/2 inch above T7. T5 is about one inch above T7. So, females should be able to touch about one inch higher than the bottom tip of the shoulder blade with their thumb, males, about half an inch.

Motion: shoulder *external* rotation
Minimum flexibility: 72° for males
                             78° for females

Note: To check external rotation, lie on your back with your arm at your side. Now bend your elbow so that your fingers are pointing to the ceiling. Keeping your elbow in place, roll your hand out to your side. The above picture shows 90° of external rotation. Get the help of an observer if needed.

So there you have it, some good, evidence-based, minimum standards you can use as a guideline to shoot for. Once you've met the minimum standards, it's up to you to decide if you need to keep stretching. If your shoulder is feeling fine and you have enough motion to do your day-to-day activities without difficulty, then stretching one to two times a week should be enough to insure that you keep your current level of flexibility (please note that this number comes from my *clinical experience,* rather than the research, simply because there are too few studies done in this area to arrive at an evidence-based conclusion). On the other hand, if you feel like you still have difficulty doing some activities because your shoulder is tight, or you just want more motion for certain athletic activities, simply continue stretching until you meet your goal. This would be the case, for example, where a worker does a lot of high, overhead activities and needs a bit more reach, or a baseball player who wants more external rotation for throwing the ball. Here again, after you've achieved your specific goal, I recommend stretching one to two times a week to keep your flexibility gains.

Use These Stretching Secrets To Succeed

Okay, we've talked about why optimal flexibility is essential to bulletproofing your shoulder, what can limit shoulder flexibility, and how much flexibility you should have. All that's left is, well, to show you how to get flexible!

While the shoulder is capable of literally *dozens* of different motions at varying angles, the truth is there are only four critical motions you need to work on to get an optimally functioning shoulder – the same ones we've been talking about in the last few pages. They are:

- **reaching overhead (flexion)**
- **reaching behind the back (internal rotation)**
- **reaching to the side (external rotation)**
- **reaching across the chest (horizontal adduction)**

While there are many different techniques to choose from when it comes to stretching out a tight muscle and improving these motions, by far the easiest and least complicated way is known as *the static stretch*. A static (or stationary) stretch takes a tight muscle, puts it in a lengthened position, and keeps it there for a certain period of time. For instance, if you wanted to use the static stretch technique to make your back muscles more flexible, you could simply lie on your back and pull your knees to your chest. Thus, as you are holding this position, the back muscles are being *statically stretched*. There's no bouncing, just a gentle, sustained stretch.

It sounds easy, perhaps a bit *too* easy, so you may be wondering at this point just how effective static stretching really is when it comes to making one more flexible. Well, a quick review of the stretching research pretty much lays it out straight as there are *multiple* randomized controlled trials clearly in agreement that this is a winning method. Here are the highlights...

- a study published in the journal *Physical Therapy* took 57 subjects and randomly divided them up into four groups (Bandy 1994)

- the first group held their static stretch for a length of 15 seconds, the second group for 30 seconds, and the third for 60. The fourth group (the control group) did not stretch at all.

- all three groups performed *one* stretch a day, five days a week, for six weeks

- results showed that holding a stretch for a period of 30 seconds was just as effective at increasing flexibility as holding one for 60 seconds. Also, holding a stretch for a period of 30 seconds was much more effective than holding one for 15 seconds or (of course) not stretching at all.

Hmm. Looks like if you hold a stretch for 15 seconds, it doesn't do much to make you more flexible. On the other hand, holding a stretch for 30 full seconds *does* work – and just as well as 60 seconds!

Wow. So now that we know 30 seconds seems to be the magic number, makes you wonder if doing *a bunch* of 30-second stretches would be *even better* than doing it one time a day like they did in the study...

- another randomized controlled trial done several years later (Bandy 1997) set out to research not only the optimal length of time to hold a static stretch, *but also the optimal number of times to do it*

- 93 subjects were recruited and randomly placed into one of five groups: 1) perform three 1-minute stretches; 2) perform three 30-second stretches; 3) perform a 1-minute stretch; 4) perform a 30-second stretch; or 5) do no stretching at all (the control group)

- the results? Not so surprising was the fact that all groups that stretched became more flexible than the control group that didn't stretch.

- however what *was* surprising was the finding that among the groups that did stretch, no one group became more flexible than the other!

- in other words, the researchers found that as far as trying to become more flexible, it made no difference whether the stretching time was increased from 30 to 60 seconds, OR when the frequency was changed from doing one stretch a day to doing three stretches a day

So here we have yet *another* randomized controlled trial (the kind of study that provides the highest form of proof in medicine) which is showing us once again that holding a stretch for 30 seconds is *just as effective* as holding it for 60 seconds. And to top it all off, doing the 30-second stretch *once* a day is just as good as if you did it three times!

Interestingly, other randomized controlled trials have also supported the effectiveness of the 30-second stretch done one time a day, five days a week, to make one more flexible (Bandy 1998). Fantastic!

So as the randomized controlled trials *clearly* point out, it really doesn't take a lot of time to stretch out tight muscles *if* you know how. Based on the current published stretching research, this book recommends the following guidelines for the average person needing to stretch out a tight muscle with the *static stretch technique*:

- **get into the starting position**
- **next, begin moving into the stretch position until a *gentle* stretch is felt**
- **once this position is achieved, hold for a full 30 seconds**
- **when the 30 seconds is up, *slowly* release the stretch**
- **do this one time a day, five days a week**

One last note. While it is acceptable to feel a little discomfort while doing a stretch, it is *not* okay to be in pain. Do not force yourself to get into any stretching position, and by all means, skip the stretch entirely if it makes any pain worse. On the next few pages are the stretches...

Critical Motion #1:
~Overhead Stretch~

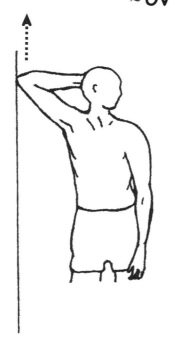

✓ Stand sideways with your elbow against a wall.
✓ Now slide your elbow straight up the wall until you feel a gentle stretch in your shoulder area.
✓ It doesn't matter what you do with your hand, just make sure it is behind your head.
✓ Hold for a full 30 seconds.
✓ Do once a day, 5 days a week.

If you can't do that, try this...

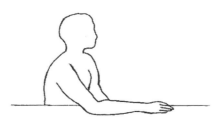

✓ Get into the above position, resting your arm on a table.

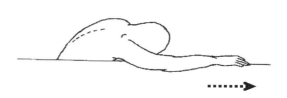

✓ Now lean forward, trying to reach out with your hand as far as you can until you feel a gentle stretch.
✓ Hold for a full 30 seconds.
✓ Do once a day, 5 days a week.

Critical Motion #2:
~Behind the Back Stretch~

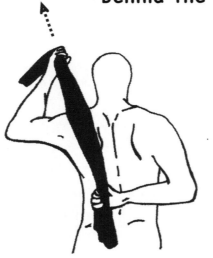

- ✓ Grab a towel and get into the position in the picture
- ✓ Slowly pull up with the top arm to stretch the bottom arm until you feel a gentle stretch.
- ✓ Hold for a full 30 seconds.
- ✓ Do once a day, 5 days a week.

If you can't do that, try this...

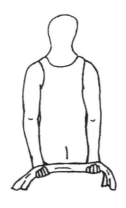

rear view of
starting position

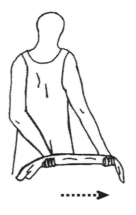

rear view of
stretch position

- ✓ Grab a towel and hold it behind your back.

- ✓ Next, pull the towel with one arm until you feel a gentle stretch with the other.
- ✓ The left shoulder is being stretched in the above picture.
- ✓ Hold for a full 30 seconds.
- ✓ Do once a day, 5 days a week.

Critical Motion #3:
~Side Stretch~

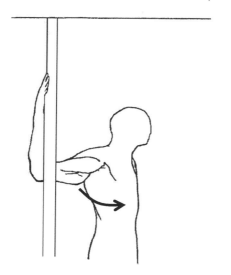

✓ Place your forearm and palm against the inside edge of a doorframe.
✓ Next, imagine your body is a column and slowly rotate your trunk away from the stationary arm until you feel a gentle stretch in your shoulder area.
✓ You do not have to take any steps while rotating your trunk.
✓ Hold for a full 30 seconds.
✓ Do once a day, 5 days a week.

If you can't do that, try this...

✓ Stand in a doorway like the picture, placing the hand/wrist in contact with the wall.
✓ Keeping your hand in place, and your elbow at a 90-degree angle, rotate your body away from your arm until you feel a gentle stretch.
✓ Hold for a full 30 seconds.
✓ Do once a day, 5 days a week.

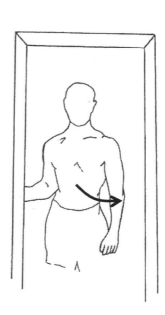

Critical Motion #4:
~Across the Chest Stretch~

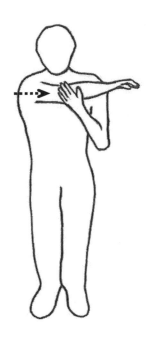

✓ Stand up straight and put your hand on your elbow as in the above picture.

✓ Now press your elbow to your chest/opposite shoulder until you feel a gentle stretch.

✓ Hold for a full 30 seconds.

✓ Do once a day, 5 days a week.

✓ We want the arm being stretched (for example the right one in the above picture) to be at about shoulder level and no higher when you do the stretch. It is okay, however, to bring the arm *below* shoulder level a bit if raising it up that high hurts.

By stretching in this manner, you are sending a signal to your muscle that it needs to elongate. Over a period of weeks, the muscle will gradually lengthen.

Pretty simple, huh? If you use the guidelines provided, stretching to lengthen the muscles of your shoulder area doesn't have to be an all-day affair. In fact, since you'll be doing a grand total of four stretches a day, it should take you approximately two minutes a day to effectively stretch! Know too, that you can use these proven, evidenced-based guidelines to do any other shoulder stretches you've found useful in the past, as well as stretches for *any other* part of the body too.

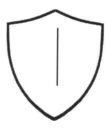

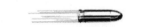

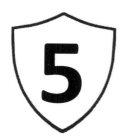

STEP FOUR: FINE TUNING PROPRIOCEPTION

Pronounced pro-pree-o-ception, all this fourteen-letter word means is the ability you have at any given moment to sense the position and movements of your body. For example, if you close your eyes, you could probably tell me without much difficulty if your elbows are bent or straight, or if your head is turned to the left or right – all without even looking.

To give you more of an idea of just how critical proprioception is, here are a few everyday activities whose success or failure depends on the proper functioning of your sense of *proprioception...*

- getting something out of your pocket
- pushing down on the gas or brake pedal in your car
- walking in the dark
- scratching that hard-to-reach spot on your back

As you can see, all of these activities involve doing something without the help of your vision. By giving your brain constant updates as to the position of your body parts, your proprioception helps you out a lot when you are unable to see exactly what you are doing.

Another good example of how crucial the sense of proprioception is to our day-to-day lives comes from a patient I had once who lacked proprioception in both of his legs. Unfortunately, this gentleman had a condition known as *CIPD* or *chronic inflammatory demyelinating polyneuropathy*, a rare neurological disorder involving destruction of the covering around the nerves. As his physical therapist, it was my job to get him out of bed and see how well he could walk.

The first hurdle we had to cross, getting him onto his feet, proved to be somewhat easy; we used a walker and his legs were quite strong. Walking, however, turned out to be another matter entirely. Each step was a journey into the unknown. Since his legs gave him little feedback as to where they actually were, his whole leg would begin to swing wildly in a circular motion as he desperately tried to place his foot on the floor. Even though he knew where he wanted his legs to go – and had plenty of strength to make them move, it was impractical for him to walk any meaningful distance without proprioception.

As you can see, there is much we would be unable to do without our sense of proprioception. Most readers of this book, however, will have nowhere near the kind of proprioception problems my patient had. Having proprioception problems to the degree he suffered usually occurs when one has a serious problem with his or her nervous system. Perhaps that is why proprioception exercises are usually either last on the list of treatments for shoulder problems, or are neglected entirely.

While a lot of medical professionals tend to think of proprioception problems as happening only in patients with grave neurological disorders, nothing could be farther from the truth. For instance, a quick look at the shoulder research shows us that proprioception deficits have been found frequently in people with *many* different kinds of shoulder problems...

- shoulders with rotator cuff pathology (Anderson 2011)

- stiff shoulders that lack normal range of motion (Yang 2010)

- unstable shoulders (Barden 2004)

- shoulders that dislocate (Smith 1989)

Apparently shoulder problems and proprioception problems can go hand-in-hand.

So we have lots of reasons to make sure that our proprioception is up to par when it comes to bulletproofing a shoulder. But in case you need one more reason, consider this:

- the shoulder with normal proprioception can send information to the brain about the arm and shoulder's position and movement in a split second. In turn, the shoulder muscles can react immediately - and contract to stabilize the joint and keep it in a safe position.

- on the other hand, the shoulder with *decreased* proprioception fails to react nearly as fast, and therefore puts the shoulder joint at risk for injury

The point here is that proprioception very much serves a *protective* role too. When the nerves in your shoulder muscles, tendons, and joint capsule immediately send feedback to your brain as to what's going on, you can then keep things under control and avoid injury. In short, proprioception helps to protect your shoulder from injury and joint damage.

A Simple Way to Work On
Improving Your Proprioception

Of all the exercises in this book this one is the most straightforward and requires the least amount of equipment – a washcloth!

Before I show you the exercise, let me tell you how studies test proprioception - that way the exercise will make more sense to you. Now a researcher in a proprioception study might take someone with, say a rotator cuff tear, and do the following test…

- the subject's shoulders are hooked up to a sophisticated device that reliably measures the angle at which the shoulder is positioned
- the subject closes his or her eyes
- the test starts with the subject's shoulder in a starting position, such as down by their side
- the researcher then moves the subject's shoulder to a certain angle, holds it there briefly, and then returns it back to the where it was (starting position)
- the subject is then asked if he or she can move their shoulder and put it *exactly* at the same angle as the researcher did

So as you can gather, the whole point is to see if you can correctly place your shoulder in a position that it was at before. And to do this, of course, you have to have a good sense of proprioception to know where your shoulder was at.

The exercise that follows on the next page has a similar theme – reproduce the letters of the alphabet by tracing them with your hand on a table – with your eyes closed.

Proprioception Exercise

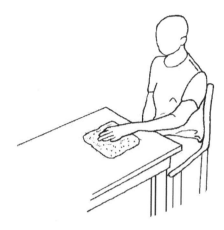

✓ Sit at a table with your hand resting on a washcloth as in the picture. Then purpose of the washcloth is to decrease friction and make your hand slide easier.

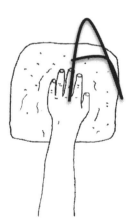

overhead view of hand on table

✓ With your eyes closed, trace the letters of the alphabet with your hand.

✓ The example shows the hand about to trace a large "A". After "A", move on to "B", and so on.

✓ It is recommended to go through the entire alphabet once a day, three days a week (every other day).

✓ It is also recommended to trace large letters, as this makes your shoulder joint move through a wider range of motion.

Pretty simple, huh? Other things you can do to improve shoulder proprioception while sitting at a table involve placing an object (say a plastic salt shaker) out in front of you at various spots (say out and to the left) – and then closing your eyes and see if you can accurately grab it on the first try.

One final note on proprioception. The research is not only telling us that people with shoulder problems can have impaired proprioception, but also that it *can* be improved with exercise. Case in point...

- this study took subjects and randomly divided them into three groups (Rogol 1998)

- group one did push ups

- group two did a dumbbell press exercise on their back

- group three (the control) did no exercise at all

- after 6-weeks, the subjects who exercised showed improved shoulder proprioception

- the control group did not improve their proprioception at all

---

So proprioception *is* definitively something you can fine-tune. And, as this study shows, even something simple as lifting weights can increase your shoulder proprioception – which means that not only do the strengthening exercises in Chapters 2 and 3 improve shoulder strength, they'll also improve your proprioception as well!

THE BULLETPROOF SHOULDER PROGRAM

The first chapter of this book explained the idea of the *bulletproof shoulder* - a shoulder that is *pain-free* and *resistant to injury*. It put forth the principle that, shoulder pain is the result of something not functioning properly, and that if the function is restored, the pain will go away. Likewise, improving shoulder function also has the added benefit of making the shoulder more resistant to injury. Then we addressed the four specific shoulder functions that need to be optimized. As you'll recall, we called them "the four abilities." They are as follows...

- ✓ **Superior Joint Stability**
- ✓ **A Rock-Solid Base**
- ✓ **Optimal Flexibility**
- ✓ **Finely-Tuned Proprioception**

The rest of the book then provided you with the tools you need in order to restore and optimize these four abilities, as well as the scientific rationale for using them. In this chapter, we will put all this information together and put it into action.

The Master Plan

This section will help you organize all of the exercises from the preceeding chapters into an easy and practical program, **THE BULLETPROOF SHOULDER PROGRAM**. Let's start with an overview of a recommended schedule for you to follow.

DO THESE EXERCISES ON MONDAY, WEDNESDAY, and FRIDAY

Shoulder Joint Stabilization Exercises

Sidelying Abduction

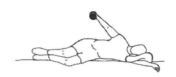

1 set x 10-20 reps

Sidelying External Rotation

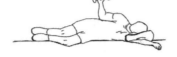

1 set x 10-20 reps

Lift Off

1 set x 10-20 reps

Scapular Stabilization Exercise

Rowing

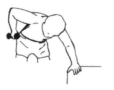

1 set x 10-20 reps

Proprioception Exercise

1 x day

Stretching Exercises

Overhead Stretch

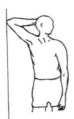

hold for
30 sec. x 1

Behind the Back Stretch

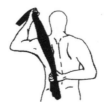

hold for
30 sec. x 1

Side Stretch

hold for
30 sec. x 1

Across the Chest Stretch

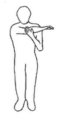

hold for
30 sec. x 1

DO THESE EXERCISES ON TUESDAY and THURSDAY

Stretching Exercises

| Overhead Stretch | Behind the Back Stretch | Side Stretch | Across the Chest Stretch |

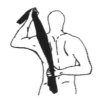 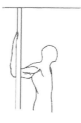 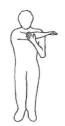

hold for
30 sec. x 1

hold for
30 sec. x 1

hold for
30 sec. x 1

hold for
30 sec. x 1

Getting Started

So how exactly do you go about getting started on this plan to bulletproof your shoulder? Here area a few suggestions...

- First get an okay from your doctor to make sure that the exercises are safe for you to do.

- Next, take a look at the weekly exercise schedule on pages 70 and 71 (the two previous pages).

- Pick a day of the week on which to start.

- Once you've decided when you'll begin, review the detailed breakdown of exercises for that particular day to learn what exercises to do. If you need more detail on how to do any of them, review Chapters 2 through 5 for more extensive instructions.

- On the day you've chosen, jump right in and take the first step toward getting a bulletproof shoulder!

What to Expect

When I give an exercise program to a patient, they usually want to know how long it will take before they start seeing results. The answer lies in how long it takes the body to adapt to the type of exercises I have given.   In this book, there are three main types of exercises: strengthening exercises, stretching exercises, and proprioception exercises. As such, there are many published studies showing that your average person can see measurable increases in each of these areas (strength, flexibility, and proprioception) *in a 6-week time frame*. Therefore, I would encourage every reader to do **THE BULLETPROOF SHOULDER PROGRAM** for at least a full 6-weeks to see highly significant gains of strength, flexibility, and proprioception in your shoulder area – as well as a decrease in any shoulder pain you might be experiencing

Now if you've seen good progress in 6-weeks' time, but you're still not quite where you want to be, continue with the program until you reach your goal. As long as you continue to do the stretches using a thirty-second hold, and increase the weight when you can do 20 reps in good form, you should see progress.

On the other hand, if your shoulder is feeling and working great after six-weeks, try doing the strengthening, stretching, and proprioception exercises one time a week for maintenance, and see how that goes. Make sure that you are using the same weight you've worked up to for once-a-week maintenance, and continue holding the stretches for thirty seconds.

Interestingly, the research shows us that it takes only a fraction of the effort to *keep* muscles strong, than it took to get them that way. For instance, one randomized controlled took a group of subjects and had them do rotator cuff exercises three times a week for a total of twelve weeks (McCarrick, 2000).

With subject's rotator cuff muscles now a lot stronger at the end of the training period, investigators then set out to determine exactly how many times a week subjects would have to do their exercises in order to *keep* their newly gained strength. So, subjects were then randomly assigned to doing their rotator cuff exercises either twice a week, once a week, or not at all - for *another* twelve-week period.

Well, at the end of this "reduced" training period, researchers re-checked everybody's rotator cuff strength, and found that those subjects who trained at a frequency of one or two times a week showed *no* strength losses. Therefore, according to this study, if one has reached their goal and doesn't need to progress any further, all they need to do is exercise once a week to keep their strength gains – *as long as they are exercising at the same level of intensity each time.*

As a practical example of this, let's say that you worked up to twenty repetitions using a seven-pound dumbbell with the sidelying abduction exercise. Your shoulder feels great, you can do what you need to do, and you have no need to strengthen it any further. So, since your "ending" weight and repetitions is using a seven-pound dumbbell for twenty repetitions, you will need to continue lifting a seven-pound dumbbell for twenty repetitions, once a week, in order to keep the intensity up and preserve your hard-earned strength gains.

Note that you will *not* maintain your strength, for example, by doing *fifteen* repetitions with a seven-pound dumbbell, or for that matter, doing twenty repetitions with a *five*-pound dumbbell. Anything less than seven pounds for twenty repetitions is a *decrease* in intensity to your muscles – and if they don't have to do as much, they will certainly lose some strength. And for goodness sakes, don't let all your hard-earned strength go to waste!

A Final Note

The first exercise program I ever wrote for publication was in my book, *The Multifidus Back Pain Solution*. It consisted of three exercises, and I asked the reader to choose only *one*. The exercises were shown to be effective in randomized controlled trials, and if the diligent reader truly followed my specific, evidence-based guidelines, I could all but guarantee that their back pain would improve, if not go away altogether.

Eventually the book was translated into other languages, and as its popularity grew, I started getting some interesting feedback from worldwide readers. Two points consistently came up regarding the exercise routine:

- there weren't enough exercises in the book
- some of the exercises were too simple or they
  were ones that readers had already seen/done before

In case some of these same issues bother you as you reviewed the exercise routine in this chapter, I would like to take a moment out to dispel a few common misconceptions before you get started. The first one is that some people think you have to spend a lot of time doing a lot of exercises in order to get stronger and pain-free – which is simply untrue. If your exercise program is targeting the *correct* problem with *effective* exercises, then you should not be spending all day doing dozens of exercises. Of course there are exceptions, but they are few.

Another misconception is that simple, uncomplicated exercises are ineffective. Take stretching for example. Pulling your arm across your chest, and holding it there for a mere thirty-seconds, once a day, may appear to some readers to be too simple a maneuver, or too short a time frame to ever stretch out a tight muscle. But on the contrary, multiple randomized controlled trials have consistently pointed out that stretching for a longer period of time, or more times a day, will not produce better results.

And finally, the last common misconception deals with not trying an exercise because, "I've done that one before and it didn't help." The interesting thing I've noted is that when you question someone carefully about what they actually did, you often find that while a person may in fact have been doing an exercise correctly, they have *not* been following proper evidence-based guidelines. Using stretching as an example again, let's say that a person tries a particular stretch that is indeed targeting the correct tight muscle, only they've been holding the stretch for fifteen-seconds, instead of the proven thirty-seconds.

After getting poor results for a period of time, most people will usually abandon the exercise and think, "That stretch didn't work." The truth, however, is that they really were doing a helpful exercise, it's just that they weren't following the correct evidence-based guidelines to make the exercise effective.

The moral? When proceeding with **THE BULLETPROOF SHOULDER PROGRAM**, make sure that you do the exercises *exactly* as instructed, even if you've tried some of them before, or they seem too simple to be effective. Then and only then can you say with certainty that the exercises in this book were really useful or not.

COMPREHENSIVE LIST OF SUPPORTING REFERENCES

It's true! All the information in this book is based on randomized controlled trials and scientific studies that have been published in peer-reviewed journals. Since I know there are readers out there like myself that like to actually check out the information for themselves, I've included the references for *every* study I have cited in this book...

CHAPTER 1

Girish G, et al. Ultrasound of the shoulder: asymptomatic findings in men. *AJR* 2011;197:W713-W719.

Keener J, et al.   Proximal humeral migration in shoulders with symptomatic and asymptomatic rotator cuff tears. *Journal of Bone and Joint Surgery* 2009;91:1405-13.

Kim H, et al. Shoulder strength in asymptomatic individuals with intact compared with torn rotator cuffs. *Journal of Bone and Joint Surgery* 2009;91:289-96.

Needell S, et al. MR imaging of the rotator cuff: peritendinous and bone abnormalities in an asymptomatic population. *AJR* 1996;166:863-867.

Sher J, et al.   Abnormal findings on magnetic resonance images of asymptomatic shoulders.   *Journal of Bone and Joint Surgery* 1995;77A:10-15.

Tempelhof S, et al. Age-related prevalence of rotator cuff tears in asymptomatic shoulders. *J Elbow Surgery* 1999;8:296-9.

CHAPTER 2

Andersen L, et al. Muscle activation and perceived loading during rehabilitation exercises: comparison of dumbbells and elastic resistance. *Physical Therapy* 2010;90:538-549.

Ballantyne B, et al. Electromyographic activity of selected shoulder muscles in commonly used therapeutic exercises. *Physical Therapy* 1993;73:668-682.

Berger R, et. al. Effect of various repetitive rates in weight training on improvements in strength and endurance. *J Assoc Phys Mental Rehabil* 1966;20:205-207.

Braith R, et. al. Comparison of 2 vs 3 days/week of variable resistance training during 10- and 18- week programs. *Int J Sports Med* 1989;10:450-454.

Carroll T, et. al. Resistance training frequency: strength and myosin heavy chain responses to two and three bouts per week. *Eur J Appl Physiol* 1998;78:270-275.

David G, et al. EMG and strength correlates of selected shoulder muscles during rotations of the glenohumeral joint. *Clinical Biomechanics* 2000;15:95-102.

Day A, et al. The stabilizing role of the rotator cuff at the shoulder – responses to external perturbations. *Clinical Biomechanics* 2012;27:551-556.

DeMichele P, et. al. Isometric torso rotation strength: effect of training frequency on its development. *Arch Phys Med Rehabil* 1997;78:64-69.

Deutsch A, et. al. Radiologic measurement of superior displacement of the humeral humeral head in impingement syndrome. *J Shoulder Elbow Surgery* 1996;5:186-93.

Esquivel A, et al. High and low volume resistance training and vascular function. *Int J of Sports Med* 2007;28:217-221.

Greis P, et al. Validation of the lift-off test and analysis of subscapularis activity during maximal internal rotation. *The American Journal of Sports Medicine* 1996;24:589-593.

Hass C, et. al. Single versus multiple sets in long-term recreational weightlifters. *Medicine and Science in Sports and Exercise* 2000;32:235-242.

Hintermeister R, et al. Electromyographic activity and applied load during shoulder rehabilitation exercises using elastic resistance. *The American Journal of Sports Medicine* 1998;26:210-220.

Horrigan J, et. al. Magnetic resonance imaging evaluation of muscle usage associated with three exercises for rotator cuff rehabilitation. *Medicine and Science in Sports and Exercise* 1999;31:1361-1366.

Kelly B, et al. The manual muscle examination for rotator cuff strength. An electromyographic investigation. *The American Journal of Sports Medicine* 1996;24:581-588.

McMahon P, et. al. Comparative electromyographic analysis of shoulder muscles during planar motions: anterior glenohumeral instability versus normal. *J Shoulder Elbow Surg* 1996;5:118-23.

O'Shea P. Effects of selected weight training programs on the development of strength and muscle hypertrophy. *Research Quarterly* 1966;37:95-102.

Palmieri G. Weight training and repetition speed. *Journal of Applied Sport Science Research* 1987;1:36-38.

Reid C, et. al. Weight training and strength, cardiorespiratory functioning and body composition of men. *Br J Sports Med* 1987;21:40-44.

Reinold M, et. al. Electromyographic analysis of the rotator cuff and deltoid musculature during common shoulder external rotation exercises. *Journal of Orthopaedic and Sports Physical Therapy* 2004;34:385-394.

Silvester L, et. al. The effect of variable resistance and free-weight training programs on strength and vertical jump. *Natl Strength Cond J* 1982;3:30-33.

Starkey D, et. al. Effect of resistance training volume on strength and muscle thickness. *Medicine and Science in Sports and Exercise* 1996;28:1311-1320.

Stowers T, et. al. The short-term effects of three different strength-power training methods. *Natl Strength Cond J* 1983;5:24-27.

Suenaga N, et. al. Electromyographic analysis of internal rotational motion of the shoulder in various arm positions. *J Shoulder Elbow Surg* 2003;12:501-5.

Townsend H, et. al. Electromyographic analysis of the glenohumeral muscles during a baseball rehabilitation program. *The American Journal of Sports Medicine* 1991;19:264-272.

Wickham J, et al. Quantifying 'normal' shoulder muscle activity during abduction. *Journal of Electromyography and Kinesiology* 2010;20:212-222.

Young W, Bilby G. The effect of voluntary effort to influence speed of contraction on strength, muscular power, and hypertrophy development. *J of Strength and Conditioning Research* 1993;7:172-178.

CHAPTER 3

Andersen C, et al. Scapular muscle activity from selected strengthening exercises performed at low and high intensities. *Journal of Strength and Conditioning Research* 2012;26:2408-2416.

Faria C, et al. Comparisons of electromyographic activity of scapular muscles between elevation and lowering of the arms. *Physiotherapy Theory and Practice* 2008;24:360-371.

Lin J, et al. Functional activity characteristics of individuals with shoulder dysfunctions. *Journal of Electromyography and Kinesiology* 2005;15:576-586.

McClure P, et al. Shoulder function and 3-dimensional scapular kinematics in people with and without shoulder impingement syndrome. *Physical Therapy* 2006;86:1075-1090.

McMahon P, et. al. Comparative electromyographic analysis of shoulder muscles during planar motions: anterior glenohumeral instability versus normal. *J Shoulder Elbow Surg* 1996;5:118-23.

Moseley J, et. al. EMG analysis of the scapular muscles during a shoulder rehabilitation program. *American Journal of Sports Medicine* 1992;20:128-134.

Ogston J, et al. Differences in 3-dimensional shoulder kinematics between persons with multidirectional instability and asymptomatic controls. *The American Journal of Sports Medicine* 2007;35:1361-1370.

Paletta G, et al. Shoulder kinematics with two-plane x-ray evaluation in patients with anterior instability or rotator cuff tearing. *J Shoulder Elbow Surg* 1997;6:516-27.

Parry J, et al. Shoulder- and back-muscle activation during shoulder abduction and flexion using a bodyblade pro versus dumbbells. *Journal of Sport Rehabilitation* 2012;21:266-272.

Schachter A, et al Electromyographic activity of selected scapular stabilizers during glenohumeral internal and external rotation contractions. *J Shoulder Elbow Surg* 2010;19:884-890.

Wickham J, et al. Quantifying 'normal' shoulder muscle activity during abduction. *Journal of Electromyography and Kinesiology* 2010;20:212-222

CHAPTER 4

American Academy of Orthopaedic Surgeons 1965. *Joint motion: method of measuring and recording.* Chicago, AAOS.

Bandy W, Irion J. The effect of time on static stretch on the flexibility of the hamstring muscles. *Physical Therapy* 1994;74:845-852.

Bandy W, et. al. The effect of time and frequency of static stretching on flexibility of the hamstring muscles. *Physical Therapy* 1997;77:1090-1096.

Bandy W, et. al. The effect of static stretch and dynamic range of motion training on the flexibility of the hamstring muscles. *Journal of Orthopaedic and Sports Physical Therapy* 1998;27:295-300.

Boone DC, et. al. Normal range of motion in male subjects. *J Bone Joint Surg* 1979;61A:756.

Esch D, et. al. 1974. *Evaluation of joint motion: methods of measurement and recording.* Minneapolis: University of Minnesota Press.

Journal of the American Medical Association 1958. *A guide to the evaluation of permanent impairment of the extremities and back.* JAMA (special edition) 1.

Kapandji I. 1970. *Physiology of the Joints Vols. 1 and 2, ed. 2.* London: Churchhill Livingstone.

Matsen F, et. al. 1994. *Practical evaluation and management of the shoulder.* Philadelphia: W.B. Saunders Company (p. 6).

CHAPTER 5

Anderson V, et al. Impaired joint proprioception at higher shoulder elevations in chronic rotator cuff pathology. *Arch Phys Med Rehabil* 2011;92:1146-51.

Barden J, et al. Dynamic upper limb proprioception in multidirectional instability. *Clin Orthop* 2004;420:181-189.

Rogol I, et al. Open and closed kinetic chain exercises improve shoulder joint reposition sense equally in healthy subjects. *Journal of Athletic Training* 1998;33:315-318.

Smith R, et al. Shoulder kinesthesia after anterior glenohumeral joint dislocation. *Physical Therapy* 1989;69:106-112.

Yang J, et al. Reduced scapular muscle control and impaired shoulder joint position sense in subjects with chronic shoulder stiffness. *Journal of Electromyography and Kinesiology* 2010;20:206-211.

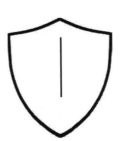